AUTOIMMUNE DISEASE CURE

A step to step guide on how to treat disease and autoimmune diseases

Dr Rowan Theo

Table of Contents

CHAPTER ONE
Autoimmune Diseases

What is an autoimmune ailment?

An autoimmune ailment is a situation wherein your immune gadget mistakenly assaults your frame.

The immune gadget commonly guards in opposition to germs like micro organism and viruses. When it senses those overseas invaders, it sends out an military of fighter cells to assault them.

Normally, the immune gadget can inform the distinction among overseas cells and your very own cells.

In an autoimmune ailment, the immune gadget errors a part of your frame, like your joints or pores and skin, as overseas. It releases proteins known as autoantibodies that assault wholesome cells.

Some autoimmune sicknesses goal best one organ. Type 1 diabetes damages the pancreas. Other sicknesses, like systemic lupus erythematosus (SLE), have an effect on the complete frame.

Why does the immune gadget assault the frame?

Doctors don't realize precisely what reasons the immune-gadget misfire. Yet a few humans are much more likely to get an autoimmune ailment than others.

girls get autoimmune sicknesses at a price of approximately 2 to at least one in comparison to men — 6.four percentage of girls vs. 2.7 percentage of men. Often the ailment begins offevolved at some stage in a woman's childbearing years (a while 15 to 44).

Some autoimmune sicknesses are extra common in sure ethnic groups. For example, lupus influences extra African-American and Hispanic humans than Caucasians.

Certain autoimmune sicknesses, like a couple of sclerosis and lupus, run in families. Not each member of the family will always have the equal ailment, however they inherit a susceptibility to an autoimmune situation.

Because the prevalence of autoimmune sicknesses is rising, researchers suspect environmental elements like infections and publicity to chemical substances or solvents may be involved.

A "Western food regimen" is any other suspected chance aspect for growing an autoimmune ailment. Eating high-fat, high-sugar, and quite processed meals is notion to be related to irritation, which may activate an immune reaction. However, this hasn't been proven.

Because of vaccines and antiseptics, youngsters these days aren't uncovered to as many germs as they had been in the past. The loss of publicity should make their immune gadget at risk of overreact to innocent substances.

BOTTOM LINE: Researchers don't realize precisely what reasons autoimmune sicknesses. Genetics, food regimen, infections, and publicity to chemical substances is probably involved.

14 common autoimmune sicknesses

There are extra than eighty exceptional autoimmune sicknesses. Here are 14 of the maximum common ones.

1. Type 1 diabetes

The pancreas produces the hormone insulin, which facilitates adjust blood sugar levels. In kind 1 diabetes mellitus, the immune gadget assaults and destroys insulin-generating cells in the pancreas.

High blood sugar outcomes can result in harm in the blood vessels, in addition to organs just like the heart, kidneys, eyes, and nerves.

2. Rheumatoid arthritis (RA)

In rheumatoid arthritis (RA), the immune gadget assaults the joints. This assault reasons redness, warmth, soreness, and stiffness in the joints.

Unlike osteoarthritis, which normally influences humans as they get older, RA can begin as early as your 30s or sooner.

3. Psoriasis/psoriatic arthritis

Skin cells commonly develop after which shed while they're now not wanted. Psoriasiscauses pores and skin cells to multiply too quickly. The more cells building up and shape infected purple patches, normally with silver-white scales of plaque at the pores and skin.

Up to 30 percentage of humans with psoriasis additionally expand swelling, stiffness, and ache of their joints. This shape of the ailment is known as psoriatic arthritis.

CHAPTER TWO

Multiple sclerosis

Multiple sclerosis (MS) damages the myelin sheath, the protecting coating that surrounds nerve cells, for your principal fearful gadget. Damage to the myelin sheath slows the transmission velocity of messages among your mind and spinal wire to and from the relaxation of your frame.

This harm can result in signs like numbness, weak spot, stability issues, and problem strolling. The ailment is available in numerous bureaucracy that development at exceptional rates. approximately

50 percentage of humans with MS want assist strolling inside 15 years after the ailment begins offevolved.

5. Systemic lupus erythematosus (SLE)

Although docs in the 1800s first defined lupus as a pores and skin ailment due to the rash it normally produces, the systemic shape, that is maximum the common, without a doubt influences many organs, along with the joints, kidneys, mind, and heart.

Joint ache, fatigue, and rashes are most of the maximum common signs.

6.   Inflammatory bowel ailment

Inflammatory bowel ailment (IBD) is a time period used to explain situations that purpose irritation in the lining of the intestinal wall. Each sort of IBD influences a exceptional a part of the GI tract.

• Crohn's ailment can inflame any a part of the GI tract, from the mouth to the anus.

• Ulcerative colitisaffects best the liner of the big gut (colon) and rectum.

7. Addison's ailment

Addison's ailment influences the adrenal glands, which produce the hormones cortisol and aldosterone in addition to androgen hormones. Having too little of cortisol can have an effect on the manner the frame makes use of and shops carbohydrates and sugar (glucose). Deficiency of aldosterone will result in sodium loss and extra potassium in the bloodstream.

Symptoms consist of weak spot, fatigue, weight loss, and coffee blood sugar.

8. Graves' ailment

Graves' ailment assaults the thyroid gland in the neck,

inflicting it to supply an excessive amount of its hormones. Thyroid hormones manage the frame's power usage, referred to as metabolism.

Having an excessive amount of those hormones revs up your frame's activities, inflicting signs like nervousness, a quick heartbeat, warmness intolerance, and weight loss.

One ability symptom of this ailment is bulging eyes, known as exophthalmos. It can arise as part of what's known as Graves' ophthalmopathy, which happens in round 30 percentage of these who've Graves' ailment.

9. Sjögren's syndrome

This situation assaults the glands that offer lubrication to the eyes and mouth. The hallmark signs of Sjögren's syndrome are dry eyes and dry mouth, however it can additionally have an effect on the joints or pores and skin.

10. Hashimoto's thyroiditis

In Hashimoto's thyroiditis, thyroid hormone manufacturing slows to a deficiency. Symptoms consist of weight gain, sensitivity to cold, fatigue, hair loss, and swelling of the thyroid (goiter).

11. Myasthenia gravis

Myasthenia gravis influences nerve impulses that assist the mind manage the muscle mass. When the conversation from nerves to muscle mass is impaired, indicators can't direct the muscle mass to contract.

The maximum common symptom is muscle weak spot that receives worse with interest and improves with relaxation. Often muscle mass that manage eye moves, eyelid opening, swallowing, and facial moves are involved.

12. Autoimmune vasculitis

Autoimmune vasculitis occurs while the immune gadget assaults blood vessels. The irritation that outcomes narrows the arteries and veins, permitting much less blood to glide thru them.

CHAPTER THREE

Pernicious anemia

This situation reasons deficiency of a protein, made with the aid of using belly lining cells, referred to as intrinsic aspect this is wanted so as for the small gut to take in nutrition B-12 from food. Without sufficient of this nutrition, one will expand an anemia, and the frame's capacity for correct DNA synthesis might be altered.

Pernicious anemia is extra common in older adults. it influences 0.1 percentage of humans in general, however almost 2 percentage of humans over age 60.

14. Celiac ailment

People with celiac ailment can't consume meals containing gluten, a protein determined in wheat, rye, and different grain products. When gluten is in the small gut, the immune gadget assaults this a part of the gastrointestinal tract and reasons irritation.

celiac ailment influences approximately 1 percentage of humans in the United States. A large range of humans have suggested gluten sensitivity, which isn't an autoimmune ailment, however could have comparable signs like diarrhea and belly ache.

Autoimmune ailment signs

The early signs of many autoimmune sicknesses are very comparable, which includes:

• fatigue

• achy muscle mass

• swelling and redness

• low-grade fever

• problem concentrating

• numbness and tingling in the arms and feet

• hair loss

• pores and skin rashes

Individual sicknesses also can have their very own precise signs. For example, kind 1 diabetes reasons intense thirst, weight loss, and fatigue. IBD reasons stomach ache, bloating, and diarrhea.

With autoimmune sicknesses like psoriasis or RA, signs might also additionally come and move. A duration of signs is known as a flare-up. A duration while the signs depart is known as remission.

BOTTOM LINE: Symptoms like fatigue, muscle aches, swelling, and redness may be symptoms and symptoms of an autoimmune ailment. Symptoms may come and move over time.

When to look a medical doctor

See a medical doctor when you have signs of an autoimmune ailment. You may want to go to a specialist, relying at the sort of ailment you've got.

• Rheumatologists deal with joint sicknesses, like rheumatoid arthritis in addition to different autoimmune sicknesses like Sjögren's syndrome and SLE.

• Gastroenterologists deal with sicknesses of the GI tract, which includes celiac and Crohn's ailment.

• Endocrinologists deal with situations of the glands, along with Graves' ailment, Hashimoto's thyroiditis, and Addison's ailment.

• Dermatologists deal with pores and skin situations, which includes psoriasis.

Tests that diagnose autoimmune sicknesses

No unmarried take a look at can diagnose maximum autoimmune sicknesses. Your medical doctor will use a aggregate of assessments and a evaluate of your signs and bodily exam to diagnose you.

The antinuclear antibody take a look at (ANA) is regularly one of the first assessments that docs use while signs recommend an autoimmune ailment. A fantastic take a look at approach you could have this sort of sicknesses, however it won't verify precisely which one you've got or when you have one for sure.

Other assessments search for particular autoantibodies produced in sure autoimmune sicknesses. Your medical doctor may do nonspecific assessments to test for the irritation those sicknesses produce in the frame.

BOTTOM LINE: A fantastic ANA blood take a look at can be

indicative of an autoimmune ailment. Your medical doctor can use your signs and different assessments to verify the diagnosis.

How are autoimmune sicknesses treated?

Treatments can't therapy autoimmune sicknesses, however they are able to manage the overactive immune reaction and produce down irritation or as a minimum lessen ache and irritation. Drugs used to deal with those situations consist of:

• nonsteroidal anti inflammatory drugs (NSAIDs), which includes ibuprofen (Motrin, Advil) and naproxen (Naprosyn)

• immune-suppressing drugs

Treatments also are to be had to alleviate signs like ache, swelling, fatigue, and pores and skin rashes.

Eating a well-balanced food regimen and getting ordinary workout may additionally assist you experience better.

BOTTOM LINE: The essential remedy for autoimmune sicknesses is with medicines that carry down irritation and calm the overactive immune reaction. Treatments also can assist relieve signs.

The backside line

More than eighty exceptional autoimmune sicknesses exist. Often their signs overlap, making them difficult to diagnose.

Autoimmune sicknesses are extra common in girls, and that they regularly run in families.

Blood assessments that search for autoantibodies can assist docs diagnose those situations. Treatments consist of medicines to calm the overactive immune reaction and produce down irritation in the frame.

THE END